Potassium Power

Beyond Bananas

BY: Valeria Ray

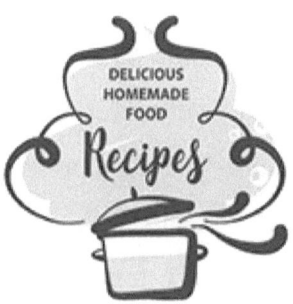

License Notes

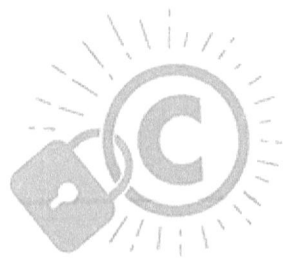

A Special Reward for Purchasing My Book!

Thank you, cherished reader, for purchasing my book and taking the time to read it. As a special reward for your decision, I would like to offer a gift of free and discounted books directly to your inbox. All you need to do is fill in the box below with your email address and name to start getting amazing offers in the comfort of your own home. You will never miss an offer because a reminder will be sent to you. Never miss a deal and get great deals without having to leave the house! Subscribe now and start saving!

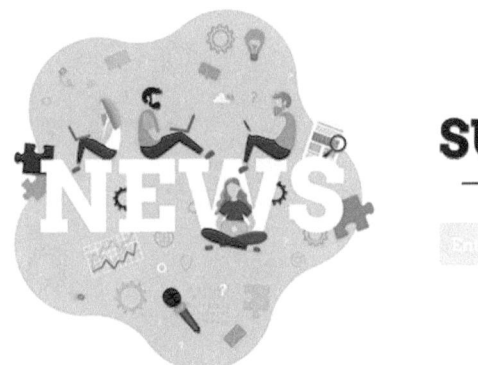

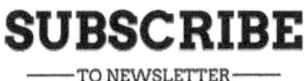

https://valeria-ray.gr8.com

Contents

Healthy Potassium Recipes

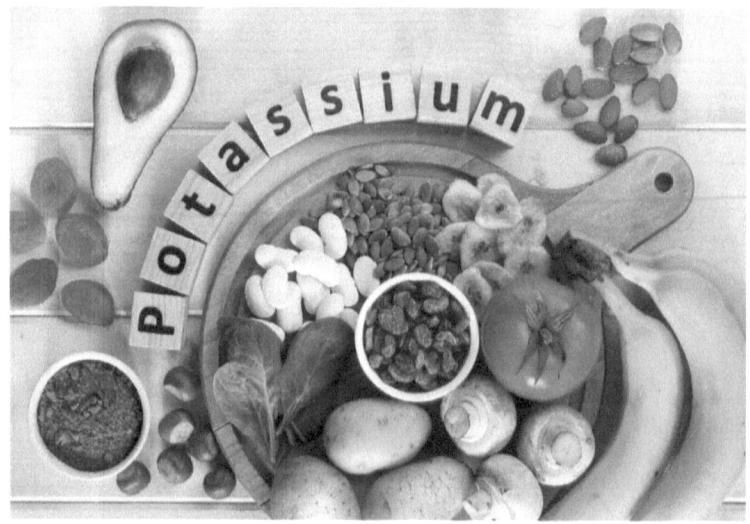

MMMMMMMMMMMMMMMMMMMMMMMMMMMMMMMMMM

(1) Pork Chops with Authentic Grape's Sauce

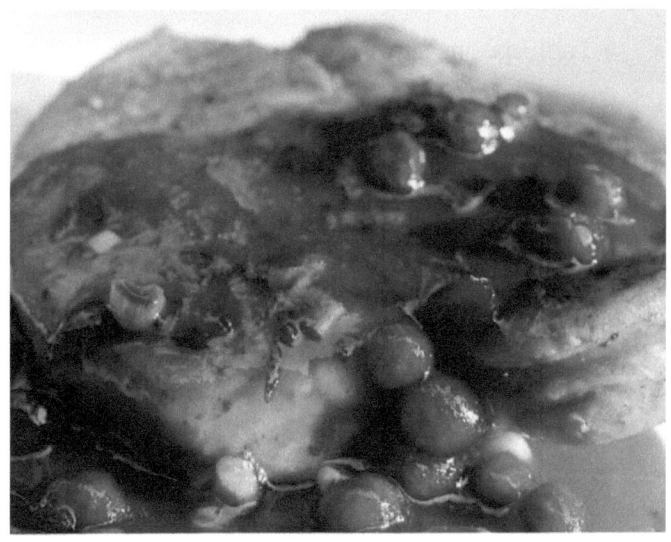

Red grapes are great for you, a great source of potassium and all. To make a very different recipe, we propose you to prepare a sauce for your pork chips. Note that this sauce recipe can certainly be served with chicken or turkey as well. This sauce has given me many compliments over the years. People do not think of using grapes on meats and they make quite delicious sauces.

Yield: 4-6

Cooking Time: 30-60 minutes

List of Ingredients:

- 4 large pork chops
- 2 cups red seedless grapes
- 4 Tablespoons white sugar
- 4 Tablespoons sherry wine
- Salt, black pepper
- 1 tablespoon white balsamic vinegar
- 1 teaspoon dried oregano
- ½ teaspoons dried thyme
- 1 tablespoon red pepper flakes
- ¼ cup water

MMMMMMMMMMMMMMMMMMMMMMMMMMMMMMMMMMMM

Instructions:

1. Preheat the oven to 400 degrees F.
2. In a saucepan, combine the following ingredients: water, sherry wine and sugar.
3. Add the grapes and bring to boil.
4. Once it is boiling reduce the temperature to medium heat.
5. Cook for at least 20 minutes. Add all the herbs and spices and the balsamic vinegar, mix again.
6. Meanwhile, in pan, sautéed the pork chops for a few minutes one each side in olive oil. Season with salt and pepper.
7. Place the pork chips in a large greased baking dish and pour all the grape sauce on top.
8. Bake in the oven for an additional 20-25 minutes.
9. Serve with a side salad or perhaps mashed potatoes.

(2) Comforting Turkey Casserole

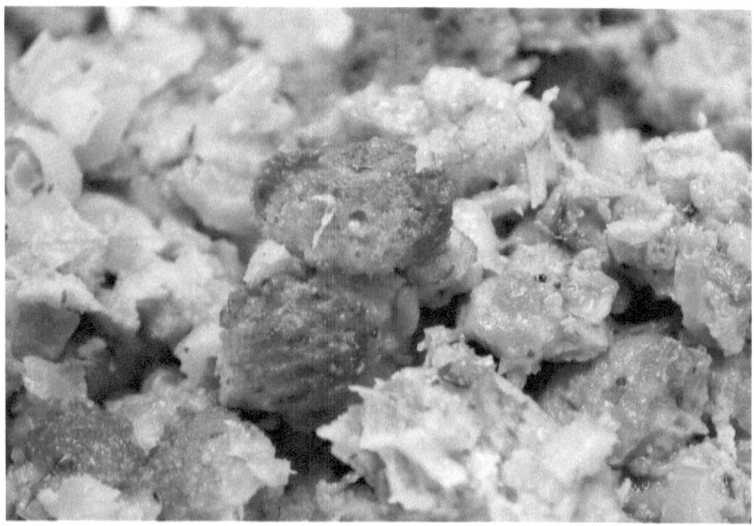

This recipe is perfect after Thanksgiving or the holidays, when you a have leftover turkey meat. Turkey is a great source of potassium and proteins and contains less fat than many other meats. Add some great veggies and you have there a very promising casserole. You can always use an additional casserole recipe. Can't you?

Yield: 4-6

Cooking Time: 30-60 minutes

List of Ingredients:

- 1 can cream of mushrooms
- 1 cup milk
- 2 cups shredded cooked turkey
- 2 cups fresh sliced mushrooms
- 2 cups baby spinach leaves
- 2 tablespoons unsalted butter
- 2 minced cloves garlic
- 1 small chopped yellow onion
- 1 large sliced peeled carrot
- Salt, black pepper
- ½ teaspoons thyme
- ½ teaspoons garlic powder
- 1 tablespoon Italian seasonings

MMMMMMMMMMMMMMMMMMMMMMMMMMMMMMM

Instructions:

1. Preheat the oven to 375 degrees F.
2. Grease a large square or rectangle dish and set aside for now.
3. In a pan, heat the butter and cook the garlic, mushrooms, sliced carrots and onions for 10-12 minutes.
4. Add the spinach and Italian seasonings and stir. Cook an additional 5 minutes. Set aside.
5. In a bowl, mix the milk and the cream of mushrooms.
6. Add the turkey, cooked veggies and all seasonings to the mixture and stir.
7. Pour this combination into the greased baking dish.
8. Bake in the oven for 30 minutes.
9. Sometimes I had a thin layer of cheese or even a layer of breadcrumbs, it's up to you!

(3) Yummy Beet Bruschetta

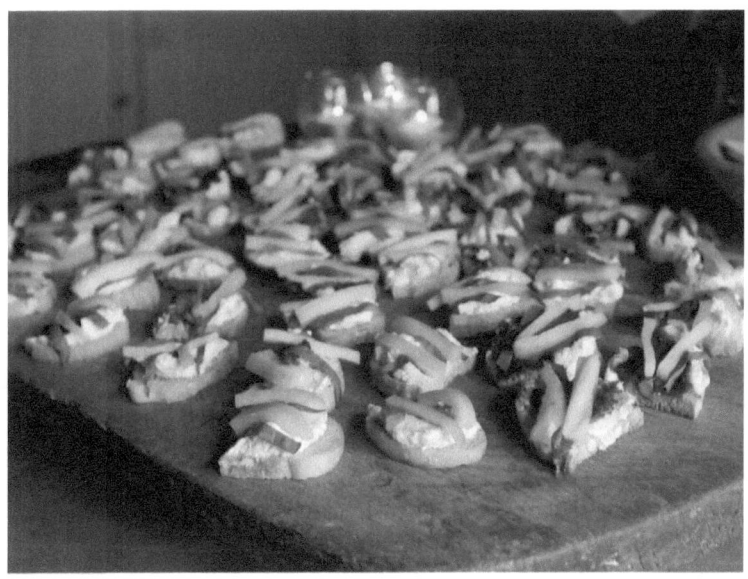

Not everyone likes beets. I like the color of it and I love to decorate many dishes with it. However, I used to never eat beets, until I realize how full of potassium they were. So, I found this very tasty appetizers recipe and now I can gobble them without any problem! You can use a flavored cream cheese, such as garlic and herbs, but I prefer to use plain, and let them beets give the special flavoring to the dish.

Yield: 4-6

Cooking Time: 30-60 minutes

List of Ingredients:

- 1 French baguette, baguette
- 3 medium sized beets – peeled
- 1 package cream cheese (room temperature)
- 1 tablespoon balsamic vinegar
- 2 Tablespoons olive oil
- 3 Tablespoons minced red onion
- Salt, black pepper
- 2 Tablespoons agave syrup
- Pinch dried tarragon

MMMMMMMMMMMMMMMMMMMMMMMMMMMMMMMMM

Instructions:

Clean and remove end of beets.

Boil water and salt and cook the beets until they have softened.

Set them aside and once they have cooled down, minced them finely.

In a mixing bowl, combine the vinegar, oil, onion, pepper, agave syrup and tarragon.

Add the minced beets and combine well.

Slice your French baguette and spread cream cheese on each slice.

Add a generous portion of the beets salad you made.

Place in the oven for just about 10 minutes.

Serve warm and perfect with a glass of white wine.

(4) Simple Avocado Salad

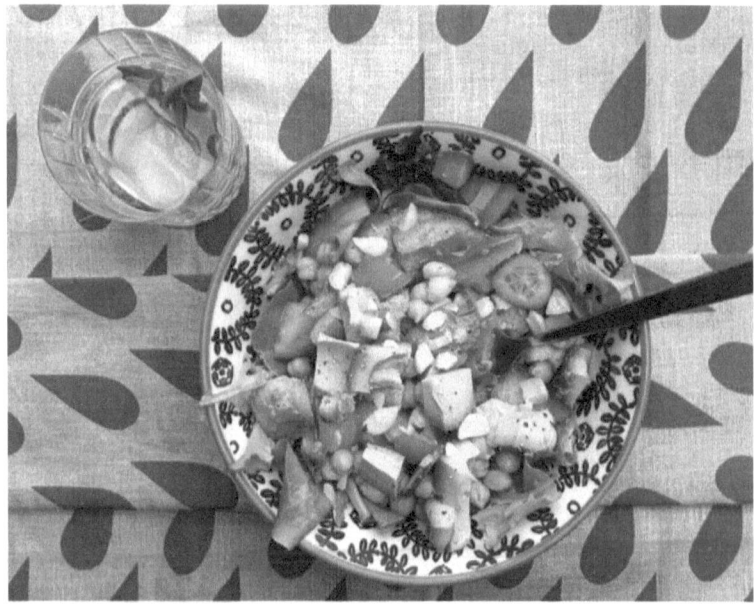

This very simple salad will give you plenty of potassium. It is also very beautiful with an eye-catching array of colors. The vinaigrette we suggest is also perfect once it sprinkled over the top, you will truly enjoy the combination of flavors.

Yield: 2

Cooking Time: 30-60 minutes

List of Ingredients:

- 6-8 cherry tomatoes (cut in halves)
- 1 large and ripped large avocado
- 1 minced green onion
- 3 Tablespoons avocado oil
- ½ ground cumin
- Pinch garlic powder
- 3 tablespoons lemon juice
- 1 tablespoon balsamic vinegar
- 1 tablespoon agave syrup
- Salt, black pepper

MMMMMMMMMMMMMMMMMMMMMMMMMMMMMMMMMM

Instructions:

1. First, prepare the vinaigrette. Use a medium mixing bowl, and combine the oil, lemon juice, vinegar, agave syrup, salt, pepper, cumin, and garlic powder.
2. Set aside and work on getting the veggie ready.
3. Diced the avocado and cut the cherry tomatoes and onion.
4. Mix them together careful and add the vinaigrette. You are all set!

(5) Apricot and Chicken Duet

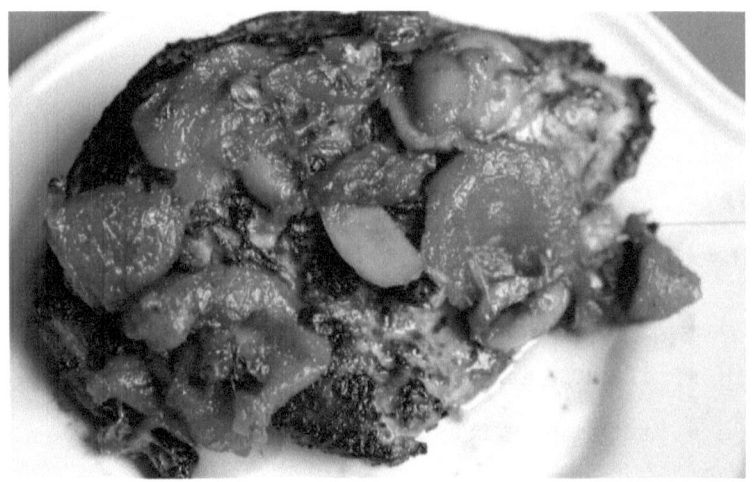

Apricots and chicken go very well together. Make sure you do add a generous portion of the sauce when you serve the chicken and turkey combination You can add some dried fruits such as raisins or cranberries to the sauce, to make this dish extra tasty and a little sweeter.

Yield: 4-6

Cooking Time: 30-60 minutes

List of Ingredients:

- 4 boneless and skinless chicken breasts
- 1 tablespoon olive oil
- 1 small chopped onion
- 1 can crushed tomatoes
- ½ cup chicken broth
- 2 minced cloves garlic
- 2 tablespoons tomato paste
- 1 tablespoon red pepper flakes
- 1 can apricots in natural juice
- Pinch nutmeg

MMMMMMMMMMMMMMMMMMMMMMMMMMMMMMMMM

Instructions:

1. Preheat the oven to 350 degrees F.
2. Grease a large baking dish and set aside for now.
3. You could very well use chicken tenders or even legs to make this recipe, it is your preference.
4. In a pan, heat the olive oil and cook the garlic can onion for 5 minutes.
5. Add the crushed tomatoes and apricot, as well as the seasonings.
6. Let the sauce simmer for at least 15 minutes and then remove from the heat.
7. Place the chicken breasts in the baking dish and pour the sauce top of them.
8. Add finally the broth and place in the oven for 40 minutes.
9. Serve with a side of rice or couscous.

(6) The Healthiest Banana Breads

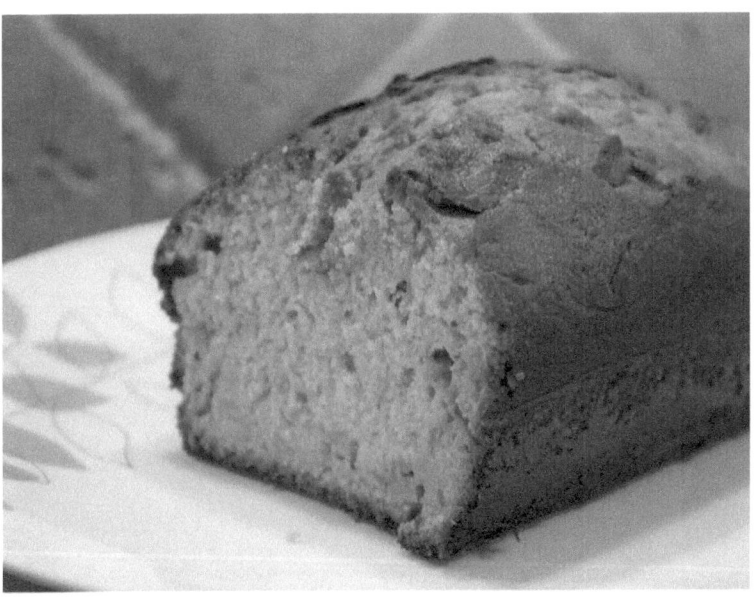

No banana bread is a bad banana bread, for sure. There are many recipes out here: some will include nuts, dried fruits, or both. You can also decide to use regular all-purpose flour or wheat, coconut flour, almond flour, or a combination of these. Let's see what this one includes!

Yield: 6-12

Cooking Time: 30-60 minutes

List of Ingredients:

- 2 large ripe bananas
- ¼ cup coconut oil
- ¼ cup coconut milk
- ½ cup light brown sugar
- 1 tablespoon almond extract
- 1 tablespoon lemon juice
- 1 cup almond flour
- 1 cup coconut flour
- 1 teaspoon baking powder
- 1 tsp cinnamon
- 1 tsp baking soda
- Pinch salt

MMMMMMMMMMMMMMMMMMMMMMMMMMMMMMMM

Instructions:

1. Preheat the oven to 375 degrees F.
2. Grease a loaf pan and then set aside.
3. Use a large mixing bowl and mash the bananas and add the lemon juice and the almond extract as well. Continue adding the rest of the wet ingredients: coconut milk and coconut oil.
4. In a different bowl, combine the dry ingredients: salt, baking soda, baking powder, brown sugar, cinnamon and flours.
5. Next, combine both mixtures together. This will consist of your batter.
6. Pour all the batter into the baking pan.
7. Bake in the oven for 40-45 minutes.
8. Serve warm or cooled down, your choice.

(7) Carrots and Parsnip Delightful Puree

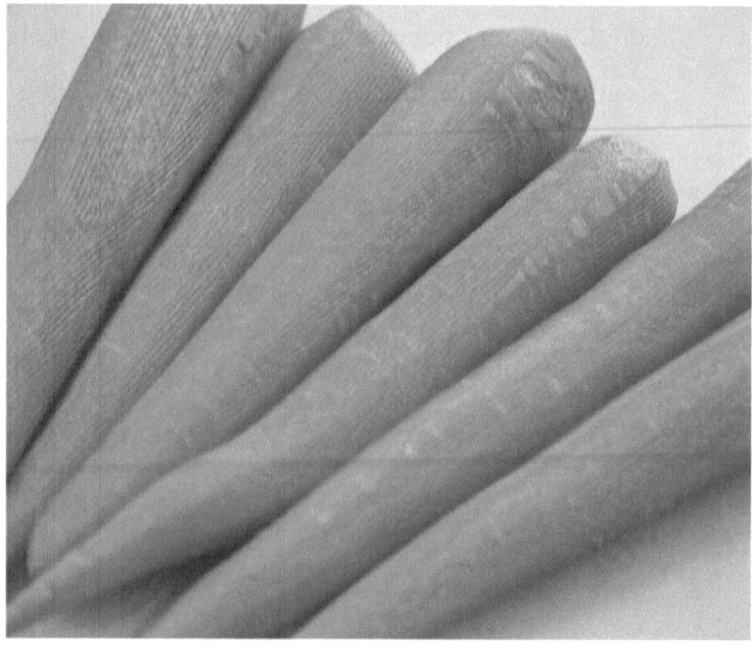

This mixture of parsnip and carrots is very nutritious, and rich in potassium. I love how I am able to sneak in some parsnip in the puree without my kid hardly noticing and get them all these very valuable additional vitamins and minerals. I have added cheese before in this recipe, but it's not necessary to be delightful.

Yield: 4-6

Cooking Time: 30-60 minutes

List of Ingredients:

- 2 large peeled and sliced carrot
- 1 medium parsnip
- 1 cup whole milk
- 2 tablespoons unsalted butter
- Salt, pepper
- Pinch nutmeg
- Pinch dried rosemary

MMMMMMMMMMMMMMMMMMMMMMMMMMMMMMMMM

Instructions:

1. Wash and peel the carrots and the parsnip. Cut in large cubes and place in boiling water in a saucepan.
2. Cook until done, it should take less than 30 minutes.
3. Place the coked veggies in a large mixing bowl.
4. Add the milk, butter, salt, pepper and other spices.
5. Use an electric mixer to reduce in a puree.
6. Serve as an awesome colorful side dish.

(8) Coconut Water Various Popsicles

Let's use the coconut water to make these yummy popsicles instead of regular water or cream or other juices. Coconut water is valuable in potassium and offer other health properties you don't want to miss out on. Make them with the kids and let them choose the fruits they want to add, that will be a fun activity.

Yield: 4-6

Cooking Time: 30-60 minutes

List of Ingredients:

- 3 cups coconut water
- 1 cup coconut milk
- 1-cup fresh diced pineapple
- 1 cup fresh blueberries or other berries
- 2 Tablespoons white sugar

MMMMMMMMMMMMMMMMMMMMMMMMMMMMMMMMMMM

Instructions:

1. Simply use a pitcher to mix the coconut water, the coconut milk and the sugar.
2. Then pour the mixture into the popsicle molds, filling them just up to the half.
3. Add some fruits in each of them.
4. Freeze for at least 3-4 hours before testing.
5. Enjoy with no guilt!

(9) White Chili for Everyone

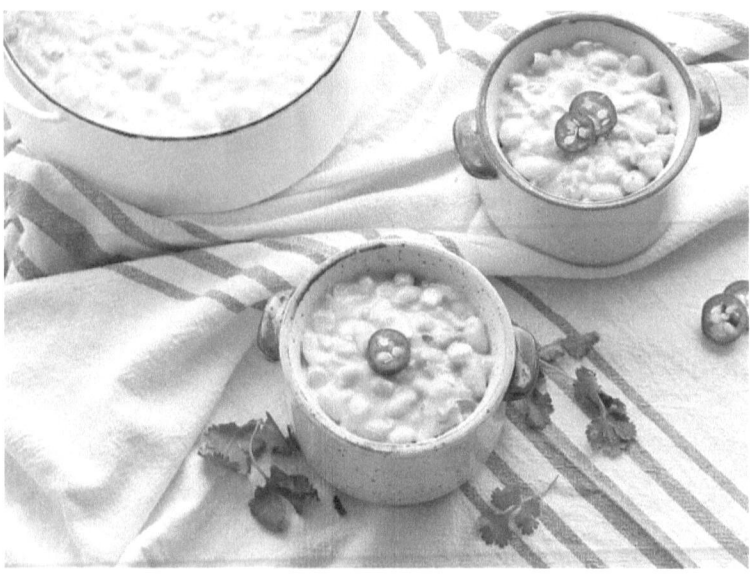

Beans are an awesome source of potassium as mentioned before. White beans, red beans, black beans, you name them. This particular recipe is using white beans and chicken, you could also opt for turkey if you prefer. Don't forget that it is easy to freeze chili.

Yield: 4-6

Cooking Time: 2 hours

List of Ingredients:

- 6 cups chicken or turkey broth
- 2 cups shredded cooked chicken
- 2 cans or about 3 cups white beans (well rinsed and drained)
- 2 minced cloves garlic
- 1 large chopped yellow onion
- 1 chopped green bell pepper
- 1 chopped leek
- ¼ cup fresh chopped mixed herbs parsley, cilantro, thyme, oregano
- 1 tablespoon olive oil
- 1 tablespoon cayenne pepper
- 1 tablespoon chili powder

MMMMMMMMMMMMMMMMMMMMMMMMMMMMMMM

Instructions:

1. In a large saucepan, heat the olive oil and cook leek, bell pepper, onion and garlic for 10 minutes.
2. Add the fresh herbs and the broth. Bring to medium-heat and keep cooking.
3. Add the white beans once you have rinsed and drained carefully.
4. Also, add the cooked chicken, and all spices.
5. Keep cooking for at least 40 minutes.
6. Serve with tortillas chips or corn bread.

(10) Classic Clam Chowder Recipe

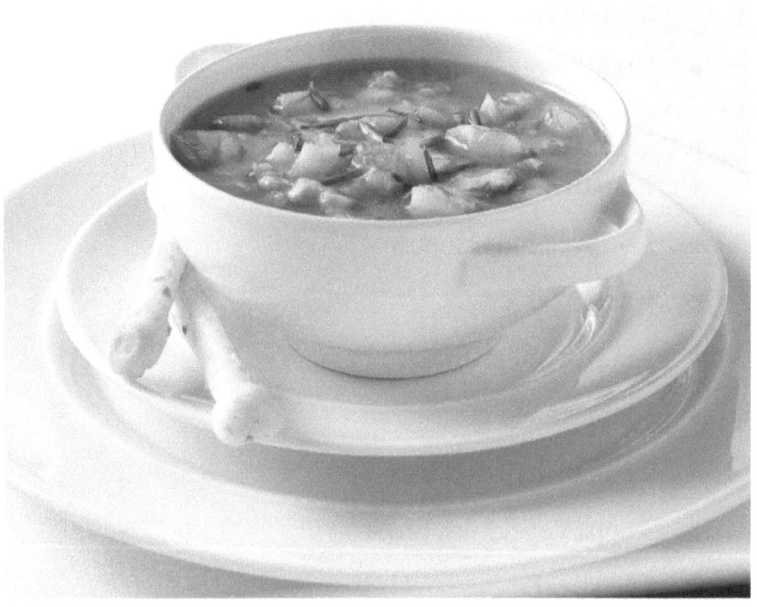

Clams are great for you and your potassium levels. Let's make some yummy clam chowder and add some potatoes as well that are also rich in that star mineral. Don't forget the fresh herbs we suggest, they really make the recipe much better. My mom used to add bacon to her clam chowder, I now decided to use prosciutto ham and I have to say, I love it!

Yield: 4-6

Cooking Time: 30-60 minutes

List of Ingredients:

- 1-pound fresh clams, scrubbed, or you can also buy them in cans, as you wish
- 1 tablespoon butter
- 2 large peeled white potatoes
- 1 small chopped yellow onion
- 2 minced cloves garlic
- 1 chopped leek
- 1 cup diced prosciutto ham
- 1 tablespoon cornstarch
- 2.5 cups half and half
- 3 cups vegetables broth
- 1 bay leaf
- 1 teaspoon dried thyme
- Salt, black pepper

MMMMMMMMMMMMMMMMMMMMMMMMMMMMMMMMM

Instructions:

1. Peel and dice the potatoes. Boil some water and salt and add the potatoes to cook until done.

2. In a large saucepan, heat the butter and coo the leek, garlic and onion for 15 minutes on low temperature.

3. Add the clams and keep cooking for another 01 minutes, add all the seasonings and herbs as well. Then add the broth and the cornstarch to get thicken. Keep cooking on medium temperature.

4. About 15 minutes before serving, add the cream and the prosciutto, turn the temperature up a little.

5. Serve hot with crackers or French bread.

(11) Roasted Acorn Squash Wedges

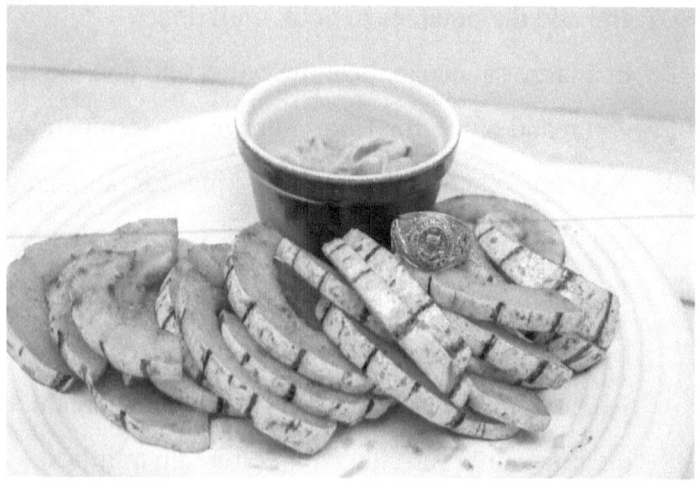

Now, yes you will get your amount of potassium by eating these delicious acorn squashes. But you will love the way the slices look when you serve them. They are beautiful, colorful and so tasty: a perfect combination!

Yield: 4-6

Cooking Time: 30-60 minutes

List of Ingredients:

- 1 or 2 acorn squashes
- 2 Tablespoons corn oil
- Salt and black pepper
- ¼ cup shredded Mozzarella cheese
- 2 Tablespoons seasoned breadcrumbs
- ½ teaspoons cumin
- ½ teaspoons thyme
- Pinch nutmeg

MMMMMMMMMMMMMMMMMMMMMMMMMMMMMMM

Instructions:

1. Preheat the oven to 400 degrees F.
2. Drizzle some corn oil on baking sheet and set aside.
3. In a bowl, mix the salt, black pepper, breadcrumbs, cumin, thyme, nutmeg.
4. Slice the acorn in thick slices.
5. Place them on the baking sheet.
6. Sprinkle the mixture of breadcrumbs and spices equally all over the slices.
7. Add a layer of Mozzarella cheese on top of the accord squash.
8. Place in the oven for 20 minutes.
9. Serve as appetizers or side dish.

(12) Spinach and Bacon Quiche

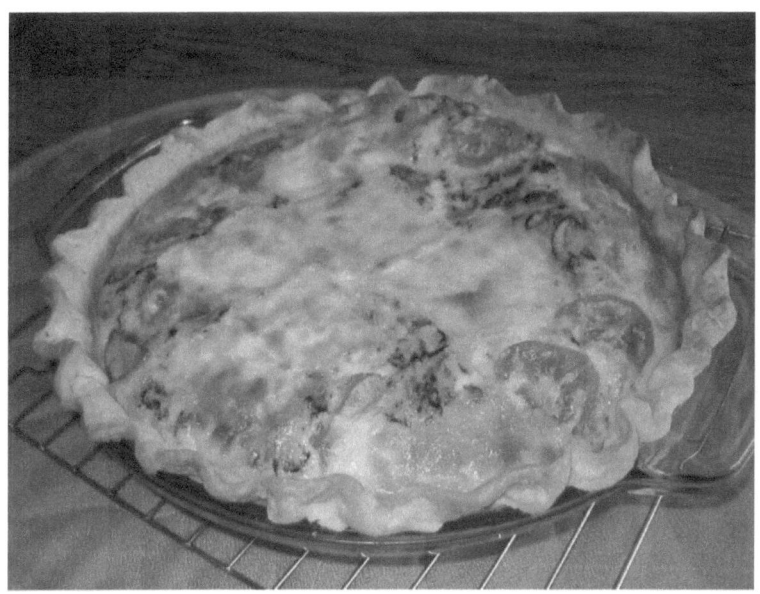

Spinach is a great source of potassium. Add it in your sandwiches, include it in salad or even r soups as well. This recipe is quite delicious, and I suggest using turkey bacon to keep the fat content lower as well. You can certainly use ricotta cheese if you don't care of cottage cheese. Make sure you do put a layer of shredded cheese on the bottom of the crust, it will make a nice cheesy crust, making it a bit different in the way it tastes overall.

Yield: 4-6

Cooking Time: 50-60 minutes

List of Ingredients:

- 2 deep pie crusts
- I cup shredded Italian cheeses mix
- 5 pieces cooked turkey bacon (crumbled)
- 2 cups cottage cheese, large curds
- 3 Tablespoons whole milk
- 1 small chopped red onion
- 3 cups fresh baby spinach leaves
- 6 large eggs
- ½ teaspoons garlic powder
- ½ tsp onion powder
- Salt, black pepper

MMMMMMMMMMMMMMMMMMMMMMMMMMMMMMMMMM

Instructions:

1. Preheat the oven to 400 degrees F.
2. You will want to sauté the spinach with onion and seasonings for 10 minutes in olive oil.
3. Do not overcook the spinach but let all the flavors combine.
4. In a large mixing bowl, whisk the eggs with the milk.
5. Add the cottage cheese, and cooked bacon and veggies and mix again.
6. Spread the cheese on the bottom of each crust.
7. Then pour the egg mixture into both crusts, equally and bake for 50 minutes.
8. Remove and slice. It is perfect served with a bed of salad of your choice.

(13) Pomegranate and Berries Shake

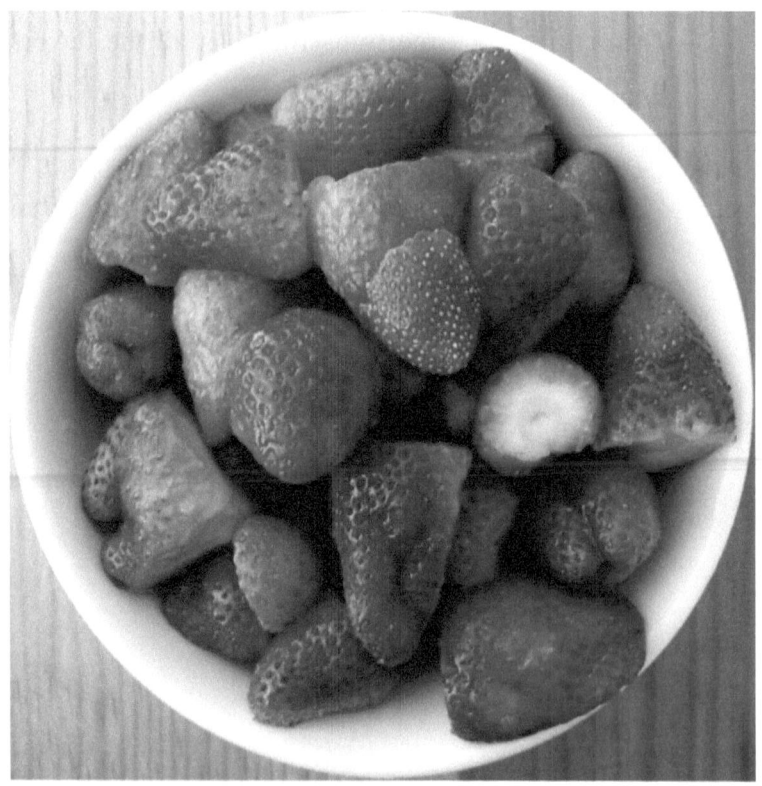

Pomegranate are very good for you and if you don't like to eat them as is, you can certainly mix them with smoothies or shakes. Also, I do suggest adding a different type of fruit also in the recipe to make the taste a little sweeter.

Yield: 2

Cooking Time: 10 minutes

List of Ingredients:

- 1 fresh pomegranate
- ½ cup fresh blueberries
- 1 tablespoon chia seeds
- 1 medium ripped banana
- 1 ½ cup almond milk
- ¼ cup ice cubes

MMMMMMMMMMMMMMMMMMMMMMMMMMMMMMMMM

Instructions:

1. First of all, wash and drain the blueberries, set aside.
2. Prepare the pomegranate by cutting the top and removing all the seeds from the inside of the fruit. Remove the membranes as well and get all the fresh from the inside out.
3. In the blender, place the fruits, the almond milk, chia seeds and ice cubes.
4. Activate the blender until the mixture is creamy and pour into 2 tall glasses. Enjoy with a straw!

(14) Roasted Potatoes Salad with Vinaigrette

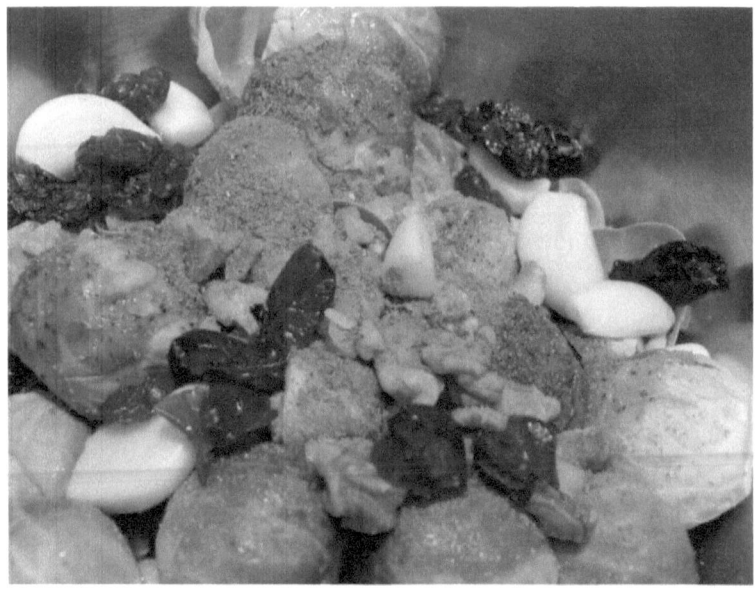

Here you go again, proposing potatoes. I suggest you keep the peel when you prepare them, as it will give you additional vitamins. You can choose to use white, yellow or red potatoes, or a combination of some of them. We will also teach you how to make this awesome vinaigrette to serve with it. I have added many different other types of toppings to this salad such as red roasted pepper or sundried tomatoes, it gives a little color, but not necessary.

Yield: 4-6

Cooking Time: 30-60 minutes

List of Ingredients:

- 2 large yellow potatoes
- 2 large red skin potatoes
- 2 large white potatoes
- 2 minced green onions
- 1 minced clove garlic
- 2 Tablespoons avocado oil
- 1 diced avocado
- 1 teaspoon cayenne pepper
- 1 teaspoon Dijon mustard
- 1 teaspoon balsamic vinegar
- Salt, black pepper

MMMMMMMMMMMMMMMMMMMMMMMMMMMMMMM

Instructions:

1. You can choose to peel or not the potatoes before boiling them.
2. I usually choose not to, unless my kids are telling me they won't eat it with the skins. But the skin contains a lot of vitamins and extra taste, so I prefer to keep it.
3. Dice the potatoes and boil them for just about 10 minutes. Do not overcook or let them get mushy.
4. In a mixing bowl, combine the avocado oil, cayenne pepper, mustard, vinegar, salt, pepper, garlic and green onions.
5. Add the cooked diced potatoes and mix well
6. When ready to serve add the diced avocado in each plate as well and perhaps a little lemon juice.

(15) Scalloped Sweet Potatoes

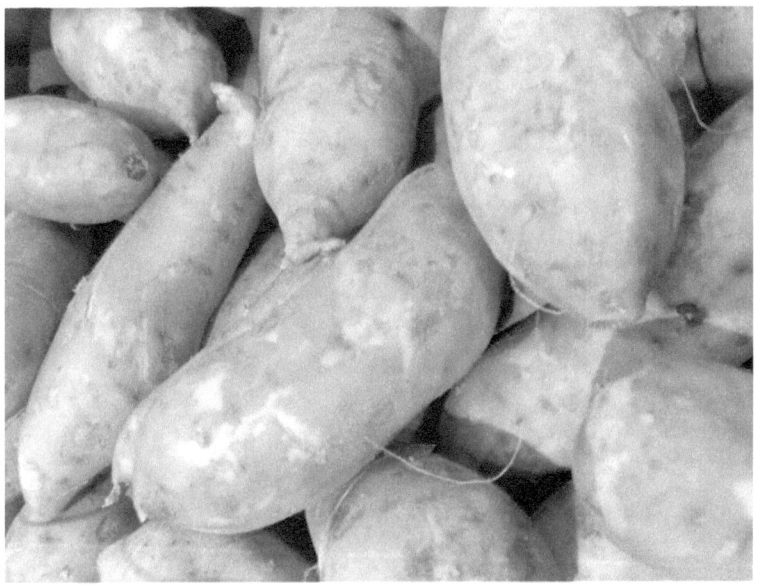

You can use sweet potatoes or regular potatoes for this recipe, they both offer you lot of potassium. The way to make sure this recipe is successful is to slice the potatoes really thin, so they can bake slowly. Also, if course the additional ingredient included in the recipe will matter. If you don't like coconut, try it with chopped pecans instead.

Yield: 4-6

Cooking Time: 30-60 minutes

List of Ingredients:

- 6 medium-large sweet potatoes
- ½ cup honey
- ¼ cup coconut oil room temperature
- ¼ roasted coconut flakes
- ¼ cup orange juice
- Pinch cinnamon
- Pinch nutmeg
- Pinch salt
- 1 tablespoon dried. rosemary

MMMMMMMMMMMMMMMMMMMMMMMMMMMMMMMM

Instructions:

1. Preheat the oven to 350 degrees F.
2. Peel and slice thinly the sweet potatoes.
3. Grease a large rectangle dish and set it aside.
4. In a bowl, mix the orange juice, coconut oil, honey, cinnamon, nutmeg, salt and rosemary.
5. Place the sweet potatoes slices into the dish as a layer, add half of the cookout oil mixture.
6. Top it off with another layer of potatoes and more oil mixture.
7. Sprinkle the coconut flakes all over the top layer.
8. Bake in the oven for 45 minutes.
9. Enjoy as a wonderful side dish.

(16) Lentils Soup in The Crockpot

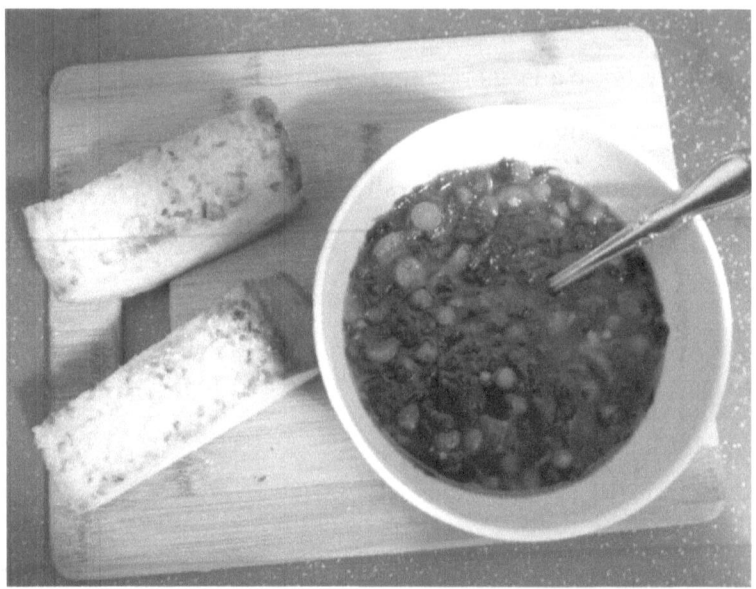

Lentils juts like other types of beans are very high in potassium. You can prepare this recipe on the stove-top or in a crockpot. I often chose the crockpot because it can cook slowly, and I can smell this authentic very healthy flavors all day cooking.

Yield: 5-8

Cooking Time: 6 hours+

List of Ingredients:

- 2 cups of dried lentils
- 4 cups chicken broth
- 4 cups vegetables broth
- 3 chopped celery stalks
- 1 medium chopped yellow onion
- 2 minced cloves garlic
- 1 large peeled and diced white potato
- 1 large sliced peeled carrot
- Salt, black pepper
- 1 teaspoon dried cumin
- 1 teaspoon chili powder
- 1 cup diced cooked ham
- 1 small can crushed tomatoes

MMMMMMMMMMMMMMMMMMMMMMMMMMMMMMMM

Instructions:

1. If you happen to have chicken bones or ham bones, please save them and use them in this soup for extra taste.
2. If not, you can still proceed.
3. Use a pan to sauté for 10 minutes the following: garlic and onion for 5 minutes in a little oil.
4. Then, add all the vegetables in the crockpot: cooked garlic, onion, celery, carrots, diced potatoes, and add both broths.
5. Add also all seasonings, the lentils sand the crushed tomatoes.
6. Turn on the slow cooker to 5 hours and mix before placing the lid on.
7. After 5 hours, add the cooked ham and cook for an additional hour.
8. Taste the soup before serving and adjust the seasonings as needed.
9. Serve with sourdough bread.

(17) Swiss Chard Just the Way We Like It

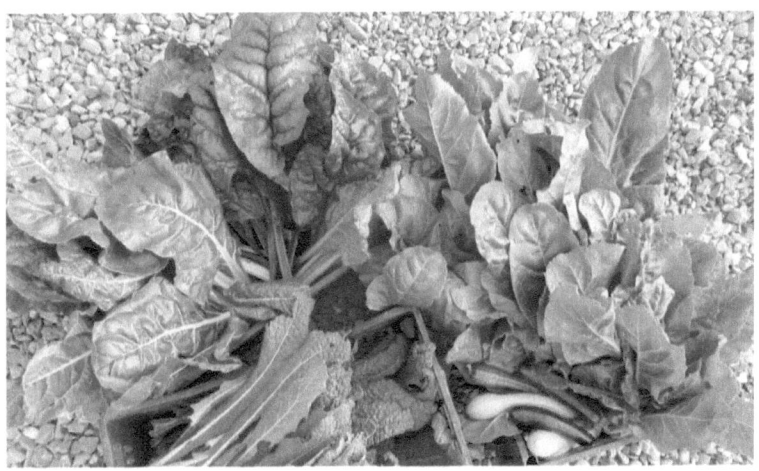

This Swiss chard is very nutritious, it is excellent source of potassium, vitamins A, C and K. It also includes other minerals such as iron, and magnesium. Also, the amount of daily fiber you will get in these greens is also exceptional, so fill up and get creative when you prepare them.

Yield: 3-4

Cooking Time: 20 minutes

List of Ingredients:

- 4-6 cups Swiss chard, fresh, washed, rinsed well
- 2 Tablespoons olive oil
- 1 tablespoon cayenne pepper
- Salt, black pepper
- ¼ cup shredded Parmesan cheese
- 2 Tablespoons sherry wine
- 2 minced cloves garlic

MMMMMMMMMMMMMMMMMMMMMMMMMMMMMMMMMMM

Instructions:

1. In a large pan, heat the olive oil and cook the garlic for minutes.
2. Add the sherry wine and the clean Swiss chard.
3. Keep cooking for 10 minutes. Season with cayenne pepper, salt, black pepper.
4. Finally, add the shredded cheese and stir again
5. Serve warm as a side dish.

(18) Slightly Fried Haddock

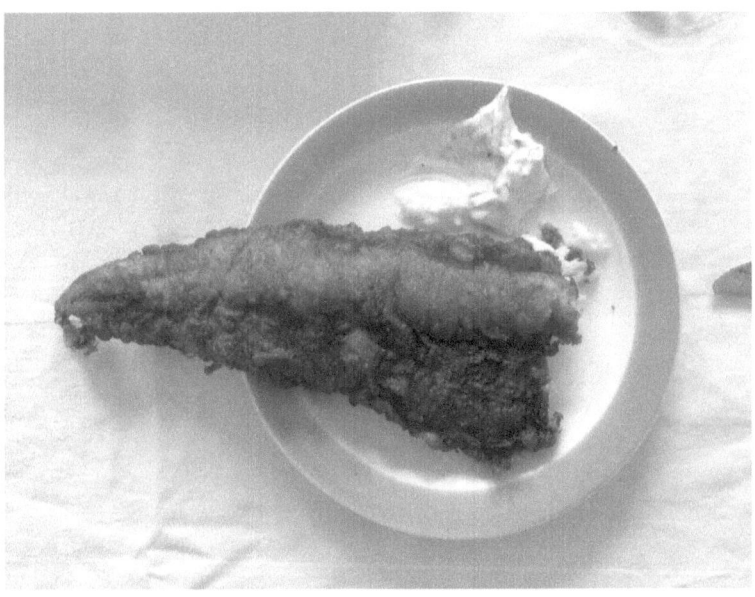

You will appreciate the taste and the nutritive value of their haddock recipe. Don't worry about frying the fish, you won't lose all the benefits as long as it is not deeply fried. Also, it is always better to eat fish slightly breaded than not at all. When serving, you can also sprinkle a few capers, if you are a fan of it.

Yield: 4-6

Cooking Time: 30-60 minutes

List of Ingredients:

- 4 medium fresh haddock fillets
- ½ cup panko breadcrumbs
- Salt, pepper
- ½ cup beer, your favorite brand
- 1 large egg
- 2 minced green onions
- 2 minced garlic cloves
- 1 tablespoon unsalted butter
- Chopped fresh parsley to decorate

MMMMMMMMMMMMMMMMMMMMMMMMMMMMMMMMMMM

Instructions:

1. Clean and arrange the haddock fillets and set aside.
2. In a mixing bowl, combine the breadcrumbs, salt, pepper.
3. In a different bowl, mix the beer with the eggs.
4. In a large frying pan, heat the butter and cook the onion and garlic.
5. Using the egg mixture, dip each fish filet in it first and then in the batter.
6. Place all 4 fillets in the pan and fry on each side for about 10 minutes or until the fish is flaky.
7. Serve with lemon wedges.

(19) Sundried Tomatoes and Herbs Rice

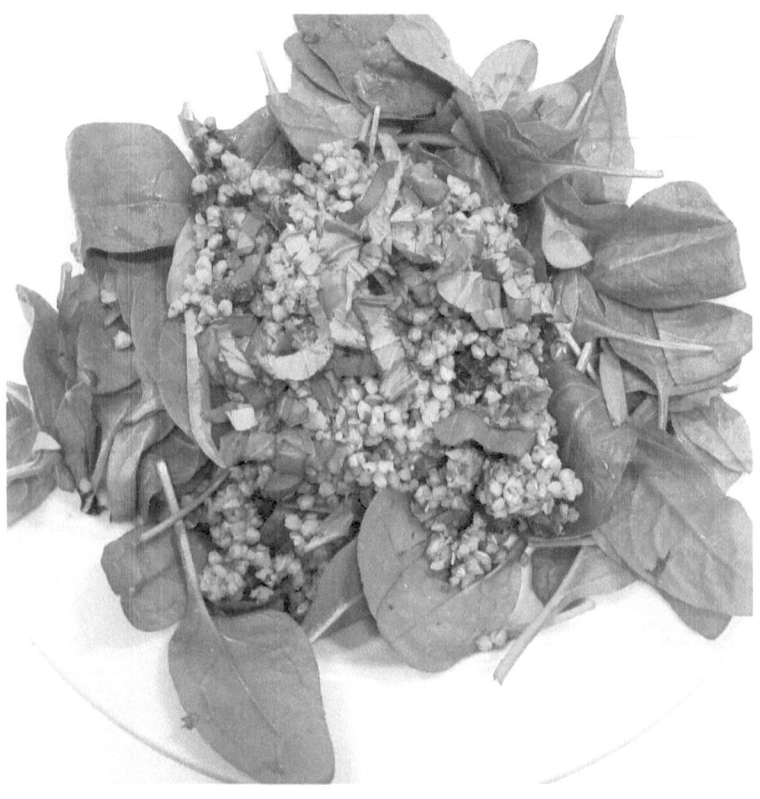

Sundried tomatoes are very tasty and certainly very pretty when added into a rice or couscous like this one. If you also decide to add some herbs or green veggies, it will be even prettier. Use your fresh herbs from your garden. You could add crumbled goat or Feta cheese also and it would be very delicious.

Yield: 3-4

Cooking Time: 40 minutes

List of Ingredients:

- ½ cup chopped sundried tomatoes
- 5 cups vegetables broth
- 21/2 cup basmati rice or jasmine rice
- ¼ cup fresh minced parsley, chives and oregano
- 2 minced cloves garlic
- 1 small chopped red onion
- 1 tablespoon unsalted butter
- Salt black pepper

MMMMMMMMMMMMMMMMMMMMMMMMMMMMMMMM

Instructions:

1. In a large saucepan, bring to broil the broth and cook the rice as you normally do or according to instructions to package.
2. In a small pan, heat the butter and cook the garlic, onion, and all herbs for 7-8 minutes.
3. Chop finely the sundried tomatoes.
4. Once the rice is cooked, add the cooked garlic, onions and herbs and also the sundried tomatoes.
5. Mix very well and add salt and pepper.
6. Taste and adjust seasoning if needed.

(20) Pumpkin Soup with A Twist

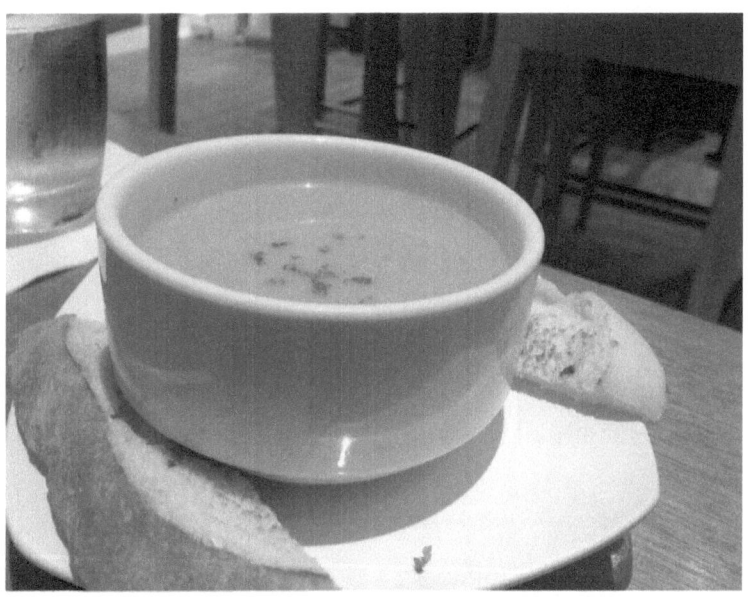

Pumpkins are full of potassium and making a wonderful soup like this one is a great idea. I like the twist we will propose while making it, because it is unexpected. The bacon is the ingredient perhaps you will not expect, but certainly appreciate. I notice that my children do love this soup, but I have to figure out if it is for the pumpkin or the bacon yet.

Yield: 4-6

Cooking Time: 30-60 minutes

List of Ingredients:

- 4 smoked bacon slices
- 1 medium chopped sweet onion
- 1 can pumpkin puree
- 1 minced clove garlic
- 2 cups half and half cream
- 1 large peeled sweet potato
- Pinch cinnamon
- 2 cups chicken or turkey broth
- Handful of roasted pumpkin seeds to decorate

MMMMMMMMMMMMMMMMMMMMMMMMMMMMMMMMMM

Instructions:

1. Cook the bacon in a pan and set aside when done.
2. In a large saucepan, heat the butter and cook the sweet onion.
3. Meanwhile, cook in the microwave the sweet potato. Peel and dice when done.
4. Add the pumpkin puree and cooked potato in a blender with e garlic.
5. Activate until you get a very smooth mixture.
6. Place back into the saucepan and add the broth and all spices.
7. Mix and also add the cream, keep on medium heat until ready to serve.
8. Serve with roasted pumpkin seeds on top. And pieces of bacon.

(21) Baked Zucchini and Parmesan Sticks

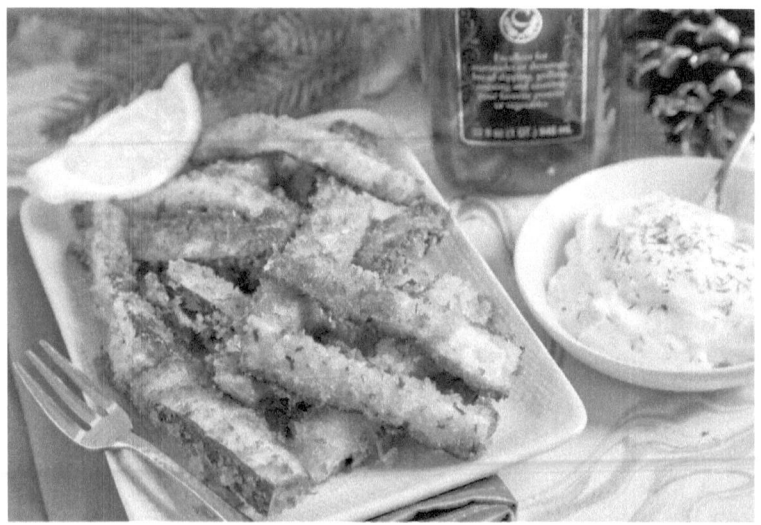

Sometimes we get tired of eating certain foods especially when some veggies have to be cooked a certain way, and that where we are happy to come in. We will make these Parmesan sticks taste fantastic and they will take you no time to prepare! Such a healthy way to serve them!

Yield: 4-6

Cooking Time: 30-60 minutes

List of Ingredients:

- 3 medium zucchinis
- Olive oil
- ½ cup shredded Parmesan cheese
- ½ cup Italian seasoned breadcrumbs
- ½ teaspoons ground cumin
- 1 teaspoon red pepper flakes

MMMMMMMMMMMMMMMMMMMMMMMMMMMMMMMMMM

Instructions:

1. Preheat the oven to 400 degrees F.
2. After washing the zucchinis carefully, use a sharp knife to slice them in 4 long sticks.
3. In a mixing bowl, combine the cheese, breadcrumbs and all seasonings.
4. Drizzle olive oil on a baking sheet.
5. Dip each zucchini stick individually in the batter and place on the baking sheet.
6. Bake in the oven for 30 -45 minutes and serve as side dish or appetizers, your choice.

(22) Gluten Free but Full of Dates Squares

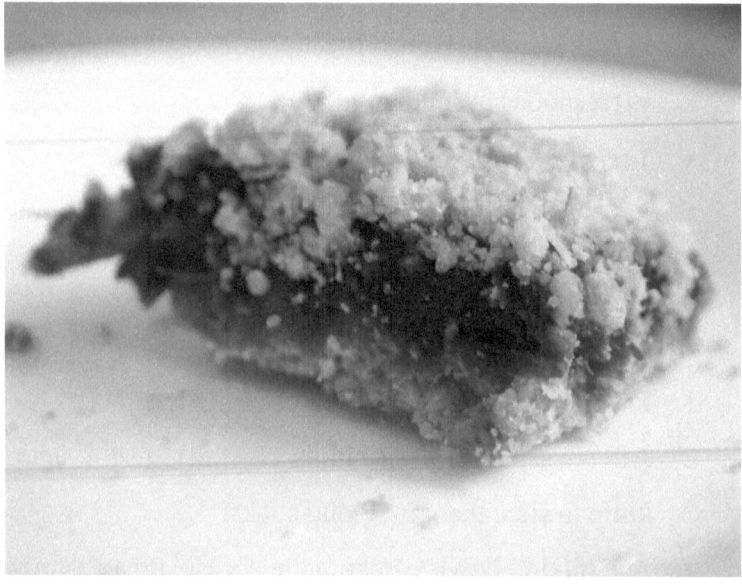

Dates are full of potassium and although sometimes I eat and serve them to my family as is, they often request for me to make the dates squares. My mom used to make dates squares when I was little, but she used oatmeal. Nothing wrong with oats, but this recipe is completely gluten free.

Yield: 4-6

Cooking Time: 30-60 minutes

List of Ingredients:

- 2 cups chopped dates
- 1 tablespoon lemon juice
- ¼ cup water
- ½ teaspoons baking soda
- ½ teaspoons baking powder
- 1 cup coconut flour
- 1 cup almond flour
- 1 cup coconut palm sugar
- Pinch salt
- 1 cup chopped walnuts

MMMMMMMMMMMMMMMMMMMMMMMMMMMMMM

Instructions:

1. Preheat the oven to 350 degrees F.
2. In a medium pot, place the dates, lemon juice, water and bring to boil.
3. Once it is boiling, reduce the heat to low and let them mixture simmer for a while.
4. Meanwhile, prepare the crust.
5. In a food processor, place the walnuts and reduce in dusty mixture.
6. Combine the nuts with the coconut and almond flours.
7. Add the coconut palm sugar and the salt, baking soda and baking powder.
8. Finally use the butter to add to the mixture to make it stick together some.
9. Use a greased square baking dish and spread a layer of the crust.
10. Add the dates mixture evenly and finish with another layer of the crust.
11. Bake in the oven for 45 minutes.
12. Let the desert cool down and cut in squares.

(23) Mainly Orange Fruit Salad

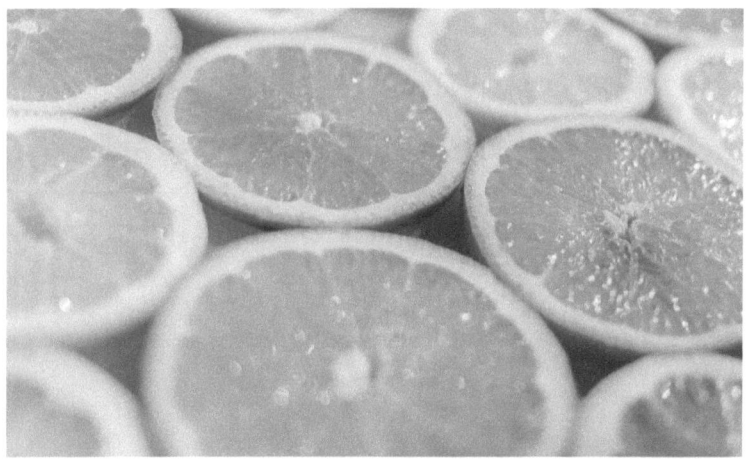

Oranges contain a high source of potassium, who would have thought? Drink it, eat it, but also incorporate it into your diet, so you can get potassium and of course the vitamin C it contains. This fruit salad will be surprisingly good and can be served as breakfast or even a side dish with a sandwich at lunch time.

Yield: 4-6

Cooking Time: 30-60 minutes

List of Ingredients:

- 4-5 fresh oranges – peeled
- 1 cup orange juice
- ½ cup pineapple juice
- 1 cup diced pineapple
- 2 medium size sliced bananas
- 1 tablespoon lemon juice

MMMMMMMMMMMMMMMMMMMMMMMMMMMMMMMMMMMM

Instructions:

1. Peel and arrange in segment all oranges.
2. Dice some fresh pineapple and slice the bananas as well next.
3. Place all the fruits into a large serving bowl and ass the juices and mix well.,
4. Serve right way or refrigerate until ready to serve.
5. You can pack this amazing refreshing salad in your kid's lunch as fruit salad, they will love it.

(24) Broccoli and Brussel Sprouts Creamy Casserole

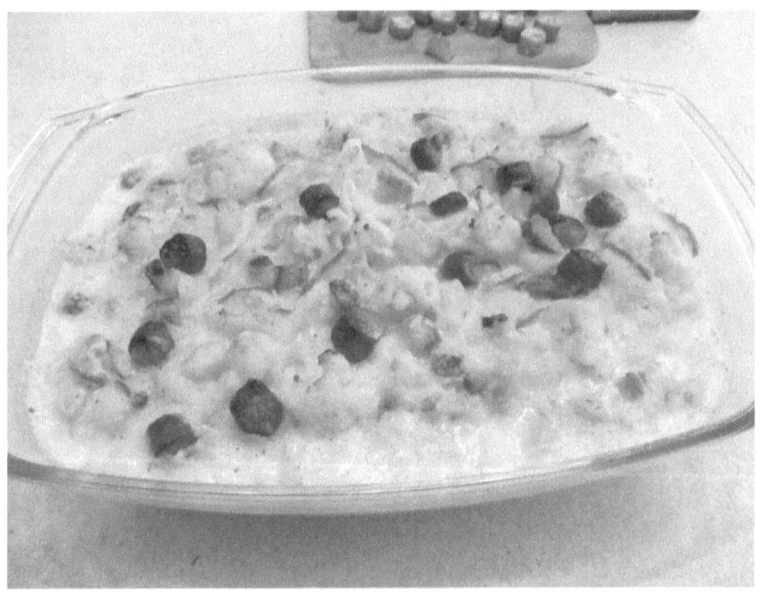

This casserole is so very nutritive. It contains Brussel sprouts and broccoli in a creamy sauce. You will love the combination of both greens and certainly the taste of the sauce it is served with, especially the cheese. Even my kids love to eat these 2 veggies now because of the overall taste!

Yield: 4-6

Cooking Time: 30-60 minutes

List of Ingredients:

- 2 cups fresh Brussel sprout
- 1 cups broccoli florets
- 2 cups whole milk
- 1 cup sour cream
- 2 cups shredded sharp Cheddar cheese
- Salt, black pepper
- ½ teaspoons nutmeg
- ½ teaspoons onion powder
- 1 tablespoon dried oregano
- Pinch cayenne pepper

MMMMMMMMMMMMMMMMMMMMMMMMMMMMMMM

Instructions:

1. Preheat the oven to 400 degrees F.
2. You need to cook the Brussel sprouts and broccoli florets ahead.
3. It will take the Brussel sprouts more time to cook then broccoli, so get a head start with them.
4. You can choose to boil water with salt and cook them on the stove-top or in the microwave, whatever you prefer. They do not to be completely soft, as they will continue cooking in the oven.
5. In a mixing bowl, combine the sour cream, the milk and the seasonings.
6. Then, take a grease rectangle dish and add the veggies and the cream mixture.
7. Combine all ingredients very well before adding a layer of Cheddar cheese on top.
8. Bake in the oven for 30 minutes.
9. Place on the table and let everyone help themselves.

(25) Appetizing Prunes Cobbler

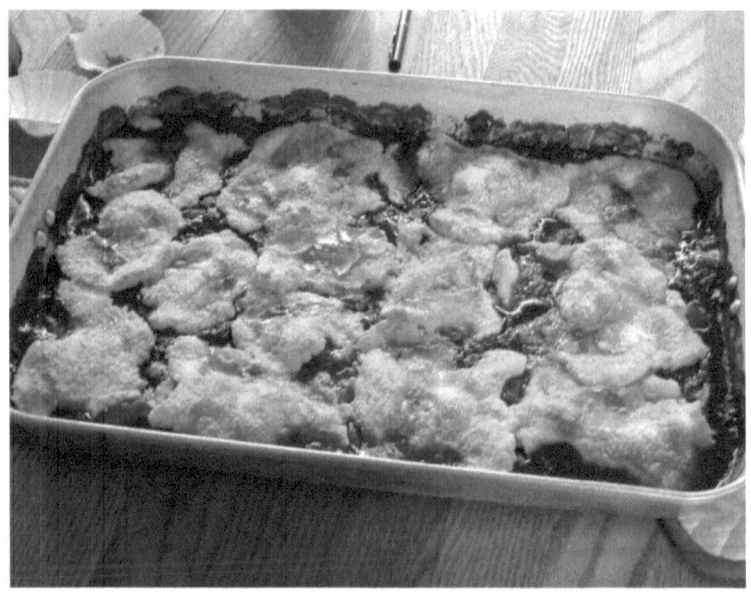

Not only are prunes awesome and filled with potassium, there are also plenty of ways they benefit your body. For a change, let's bake them and make this wonderful cobbler. You can serve this desert with plain yogurt, whipped cream or vanilla ice cream. This cobbler is certainly unique and will surprise you in a delicious way.

Yield: 4-6

Cooking Time: 30-60 minutes

List of Ingredients:

- 1-pound fresh ripped plums
- ¼ cup coconut palm sugar
- ¼ cup water
- 1 cup oats
- ½ cup all -purpose flour
- Pinch cinnamon
- Pinch salt
- 1 teaspoon baking powder
- ½ cup brown sugar
- 1 large egg
- ¼ cup coconut oil (room temperature)

MMMMMMMMMMMMMMMMMMMMMMMMMMMMMMMMM

Instructions:

1. Preheat the oven to 350 degrees F.
2. In a medium saucepan, bring to boil the following ingredients: chopped plums, water, coconut palm sugar for 5 minutes.
3. Reduce the heat and let it simmers for another 15-20 minutes.
4. Meanwhile, grease a square baking pan and set aside.
5. In a mixing bowl, combine the baking powder, brown sugar, salt cinnamon, oats and flour.
6. Add the room temperature coconut oil to it, then you have your crumbled topping.
7. Place the fruits mixture on the bottom of the baking dish and add the oats mixture on top.,
8. Bake for 30 minutes and serve warm with vanilla ice cream.

About the Author

A native of Indianapolis, Indiana, Valeria Ray found her passion for cooking while she was studying English Literature at Oakland City University. She decided to try a cooking course with her friends and the experience changed her forever. She enrolled at the Art Institute of Indiana which offered extensive courses in the culinary Arts. Once Ray dipped her toe in the cooking world, she never looked back.

When Valeria graduated, she worked in French restaurants in the Indianapolis area until she became the head chef at one of the 5-star establishments in the area. Valeria's attention to taste and visual detail caught the eye of a local business person who expressed an interest in publishing her recipes. Valeria began her secondary career authoring cookbooks and e-books which she tackled with as much talent and gusto as her first career. Her passion for food leaps off the page of her books which have colourful anecdotes and stunning pictures of dishes she has prepared herself.

Valeria Ray lives in Indianapolis with her husband of 15 years, Tom, her daughter, Isobel and their loveable Golden Retriever, Goldy. Valeria enjoys cooking special dishes in her large, comfortable kitchen where the family gets involved in preparing meals. This successful, dynamic chef is an inspiration to culinary students and novice cooks everywhere.

•••••••••••••••••••••

Author's Afterthoughts

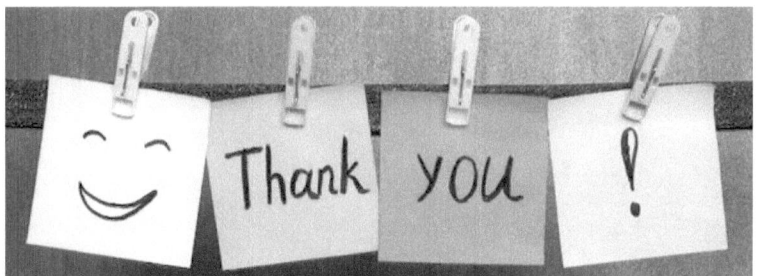

Thank you for Purchasing my book and taking the time to read it from front to back. I am always grateful when a reader chooses my work and I hope you enjoyed it!

With the vast selection available online, I am touched that you chose to be purchasing my work and take valuable time out of your life to read it. My hope is that you feel you made the right decision.

I very much would like to know what you thought of the book. Please take the time to write an honest and informative review on Amazon.com. Your experience and opinions will be of great benefit to me and those readers looking to make an informed choice.

With much thanks,

Valeria Ray